This journal belongs to

_____

_____

Address:

_____
_____
_____
_____

Emergency Contact:

_____
_____
_____
_____

Important Informations:

_____
_____
_____
_____

Date: 3-20-23   Start: 4:50 AM

Weather: Cold
         Cloudy

Water Intake: [✓][✓][✓][✓][✓]
              [ ][ ][ ][ ][ ]

Temperature:_____

Level of Pain

No Pain   0 1 2 3 4 5 6 7 8 9 10   Severe Pain

Where does it hurt?	None—Mild—Moderate—Severe			
Back mid back		X		
Head				
Neck		X		
Shoulder				
Elbow				
Buttock			X	
Knee				
Hip		X		
Back left side		X	— X	
Stomach		X	— X	

Interference of Pain on Sleep

None   0 1 2 ③ 4 5 6 7 8 9 10   Significant

Fatigue

None   0 1 2 3 4 ⑤ 6 7 8 9 10   Significant

Exercise

Daily   0 1 2 ③ 4 5 6 7 8 9 10   No Exercise
         Steps

Mood:

☺ ☺ •••
☹ ☹ ><

Food Intake:

TIME	FOOD	TRIGGERS/REACTION
8:15Am	Berry Yogurt Smothie	
11:45Am	Tuna Casserole	Reflux

Medications/Supplements

NAME	DOSAGE	TIME	SIDE EFFECTS/ COMMENTS
Robaxin		4:30	

Notes:

Stomach issues continue off and on pain mid center between ribs and belly button. Sometimes today lower center and lower mid left.

Date: 3-22-23 Start: 4:50Am

Weather: _____

Water Intake: 🥤🥤🥤🥤🥤 🥤🥤🥤🥤🥤

Temperature: Normal

Level of Pain

No Pain   0 1 2 3 4 5 6 7 8 9 10   Severe Pain

Where does it hurt?	None	Mild	Moderate	Severe
Back	☐	☐	☐	☐
Head	☐	☐	☐	☐
Neck	☐	☐	☐	☐
Shoulder	☐	☐	☐	☐
Elbow	☐	☐	☐	☐
Buttock	☐	☐	☐	☐
Knee	☐	☐	☐	☐
Hip	☐	☐	☐	☐
Stomach ache	☐	✓	☐	☐
	☐	☐	☐	☐

Interference of Pain on Sleep

None   0 1 2 3 4 5 ⑥ 7 8 9 10   Significant

Fatigue

None   0 1 2 3 4 5 ⑥ 7 8 9 10   Significant

Exercise

Daily   0 1 2 3 4 5 ⑥ 7 8 9 10   No Exercise

Mood:

Food Intake:

TIME	FOOD	TRIGGERS/REACTION

Medications/Supplements

NAME	DOSAGE	TIME	SIDE EFFECTS/ COMMENTS
Robaxin	750		
meloxicam	7.5		
Zolpidem			
Camrese			

Notes:

Date:_____   Start:_____

Weather:_____   Water Intake: ⊔⊔⊔⊔⊔
_____   ⊔⊔⊔⊔⊔

Temperature:_____   Level of Pain
_____

No Pain   0 1 2 3 4 5 6 7 8 9 10   Severe Pain

Where does it hurt?	None—Mild—Moderate—Severe			
Back	☐	☐	☐	☐
Head	☐	☐	☐	☐
Neck	☐	☐	☐	☐
Shoulder	☐	☐	☐	☐
Elbow	☐	☐	☐	☐
Buttock	☐	☐	☐	☐
Knee	☐	☐	☐	☐
Hip	☐	☐	☐	☐
	☐	☐	☐	☐
	☐	☐	☐	☐

Interference of Pain on Sleep

None   0 1 2 3 4 5 6 7 8 9 10   Significant

Fatigue

None   0 1 2 3 4 5 6 7 8 9 10   Significant

Exercise

Daily   0 1 2 3 4 5 6 7 8 9 10   No Exercise

Mood:

Food Intake:

TIME	FOOD	TRIGGERS/REACTION

Medications/Supplements

NAME	DOSAGE	TIME	SIDE EFFECTS/ COMMENTS

Notes:

Date:_____ Start:_____

Weather:_____ Water Intake: ⊽⊽⊽⊽⊽
_____ ⊽⊽⊽⊽⊽

Temperature:_____ Level of Pain
_____
No Pain   0 1 2 3 4 5 6 7 8 9 10   Severe Pain

Where does it hurt?	None—Mild—Moderate—Severe			
Back	☐	☐	☐	☐
Head	☐	☐	☐	☐
Neck	☐	☐	☐	☐
Shoulder	☐	☐	☐	☐
Elbow	☐	☐	☐	☐
Buttock	☐	☐	☐	☐
Knee	☐	☐	☐	☐
Hip	☐	☐	☐	☐
	☐	☐	☐	☐
	☐	☐	☐	☐

Interference of Pain on Sleep
_____
None   0 1 2 3 4 5 6 7 8 9 10   Significant

Fatigue
_____
None   0 1 2 3 4 5 6 7 8 9 10   Significant

Exercise
_____
Daily   0 1 2 3 4 5 6 7 8 9 10   No Exercise

Mood:
😊 🙂 😐
🙁 ☹️ 😣

Food Intake:

TIME	FOOD	TRIGGERS/REACTION

Medications/Supplements

NAME	DOSAGE	TIME	SIDE EFFECTS/ COMMENTS

Notes:

Date:_____ Start:_____

Weather:_____ Water Intake: ▽▽▽▽▽ ▽▽▽▽▽
_____

Temperature:_____ Level of Pain
_____
No Pain   0 1 2 3 4 5 6 7 8 9 10   Severe Pain

Where does it hurt?	None—Mild—Moderate—Severe
Back	☐ ☐ ☐ ☐
Head	☐ ☐ ☐ ☐
Neck	☐ ☐ ☐ ☐
Shoulder	☐ ☐ ☐ ☐
Elbow	☐ ☐ ☐ ☐
Buttock	☐ ☐ ☐ ☐
Knee	☐ ☐ ☐ ☐
Hip	☐ ☐ ☐ ☐
	☐ ☐ ☐ ☐
	☐ ☐ ☐ ☐

Interference of Pain on Sleep
_____
None   0 1 2 3 4 5 6 7 8 9 10   Significant

Mood:

Fatigue
_____
None   0 1 2 3 4 5 6 7 8 9 10   Significant

Exercise
_____
Daily   0 1 2 3 4 5 6 7 8 9 10   No Exercise

Food Intake:

TIME	FOOD	TRIGGERS/REACTION

Medications/Supplements

NAME	DOSAGE	TIME	SIDE EFFECTS/ COMMENTS

Notes:

Date:_____   Start:_____

Weather:_____   Water Intake: ▽▽▽▽▽
_____   ▽▽▽▽▽

Temperature:_____   Level of Pain
_____
                        No Pain   0 1 2 3 4 5 6 7 8 9 10   Severe Pain

Where does it hurt?	None—Mild—Moderate—Severe			
Back	☐	☐	☐	☐
Head	☐	☐	☐	☐
Neck	☐	☐	☐	☐
Shoulder	☐	☐	☐	☐
Elbow	☐	☐	☐	☐
Buttock	☐	☐	☐	☐
Knee	☐	☐	☐	☐
Hip	☐	☐	☐	☐
	☐	☐	☐	☐
	☐	☐	☐	☐

Interference of Pain on Sleep
_____
None   0 1 2 3 4 5 6 7 8 9 10   Significant   Mood:

Fatigue
_____
None   0 1 2 3 4 5 6 7 8 9 10   Significant

Exercise
_____
Daily   0 1 2 3 4 5 6 7 8 9 10   No Exercise

Food Intake:

TIME	FOOD	TRIGGERS/REACTION

Medications/Supplements

NAME	DOSAGE	TIME	SIDE EFFECTS/ COMMENTS

Notes:

Date:_____   Start:_____

Weather:_____   Water Intake: ⊔⊔⊔⊔⊔
_____   ⊔⊔⊔⊔⊔

Temperature:_____   Level of Pain
                         _____
                         No Pain   0 1 2 3 4 5 6 7 8 9 10   Severe Pain

Where does it hurt?	None—Mild—Moderate—Severe			
Back	☐	☐	☐	☐
Head	☐	☐	☐	☐
Neck	☐	☐	☐	☐
Shoulder	☐	☐	☐	☐
Elbow	☐	☐	☐	☐
Buttock	☐	☐	☐	☐
Knee	☐	☐	☐	☐
Hip	☐	☐	☐	☐
	☐	☐	☐	☐
	☐	☐	☐	☐

Interference of Pain on Sleep
_____

None   0 1 2 3 4 5 6 7 8 9 10   Significant

Fatigue
_____

None   0 1 2 3 4 5 6 7 8 9 10   Significant

Exercise
_____

Daily   0 1 2 3 4 5 6 7 8 9 10   No Exercise

Mood:

Food Intake:

TIME	FOOD	TRIGGERS/REACTION

Medications/Supplements

NAME	DOSAGE	TIME	SIDE EFFECTS/ COMMENTS

Notes:

Date:_____   Start:_____

Weather:_____   Water Intake: ⊔⊔⊔⊔⊔
_____   ⊔⊔⊔⊔⊔

Temperature:_____   Level of Pain
_____
                           No Pain   0 1 2 3 4 5 6 7 8 9 10   Severe Pain

Where does it hurt?	None—Mild—Moderate—Severe			
Back	☐	☐	☐	☐
Head	☐	☐	☐	☐
Neck	☐	☐	☐	☐
Shoulder	☐	☐	☐	☐
Elbow	☐	☐	☐	☐
Buttock	☐	☐	☐	☐
Knee	☐	☐	☐	☐
Hip	☐	☐	☐	☐
	☐	☐	☐	☐
	☐	☐	☐	☐

Interference of Pain on Sleep
_____
None   0 1 2 3 4 5 6 7 8 9 10   Significant

Fatigue
_____
None   0 1 2 3 4 5 6 7 8 9 10   Significant

Exercise
_____
Daily   0 1 2 3 4 5 6 7 8 9 10   No Exercise

Mood:

Food Intake:

TIME	FOOD	TRIGGERS/REACTION

Medications/Supplements

NAME	DOSAGE	TIME	SIDE EFFECTS/ COMMENTS

Notes:

Date:_____   Start:_____

Weather:_____   Water Intake: ▽▽▽▽▽ ▽▽▽▽▽

Temperature:_____   Level of Pain

No Pain   0 1 2 3 4 5 6 7 8 9 10   Severe Pain

Where does it hurt?	None—Mild—Moderate—Severe			
Back	☐	☐	☐	☐
Head	☐	☐	☐	☐
Neck	☐	☐	☐	☐
Shoulder	☐	☐	☐	☐
Elbow	☐	☐	☐	☐
Buttock	☐	☐	☐	☐
Knee	☐	☐	☐	☐
Hip	☐	☐	☐	☐
	☐	☐	☐	☐
	☐	☐	☐	☐

Interference of Pain on Sleep

None   0 1 2 3 4 5 6 7 8 9 10   Significant

Fatigue

None   0 1 2 3 4 5 6 7 8 9 10   Significant

Exercise

Daily   0 1 2 3 4 5 6 7 8 9 10   No Exercise

Mood:

Food Intake:

TIME	FOOD	TRIGGERS/REACTION

Medications/Supplements

NAME	DOSAGE	TIME	SIDE EFFECTS/ COMMENTS

Notes:

Date:_____   Start:_____

Weather:_____   Water Intake: ⊔⊔⊔⊔⊔
_____   ⊔⊔⊔⊔⊔

Temperature:_____   Level of Pain
                         _____
                         No Pain   0 1 2 3 4 5 6 7 8 9 10   Severe Pain

Where does it hurt?	None—Mild—Moderate—Severe			
Back	☐	☐	☐	☐
Head	☐	☐	☐	☐
Neck	☐	☐	☐	☐
Shoulder	☐	☐	☐	☐
Elbow	☐	☐	☐	☐
Buttock	☐	☐	☐	☐
Knee	☐	☐	☐	☐
Hip	☐	☐	☐	☐
	☐	☐	☐	☐
	☐	☐	☐	☐

Interference of Pain on Sleep
_____
None   0 1 2 3 4 5 6 7 8 9 10   Significant

Fatigue
_____
None   0 1 2 3 4 5 6 7 8 9 10   Significant

Exercise
_____
Daily   0 1 2 3 4 5 6 7 8 9 10   No Exercise

Mood:
😊 🙂 😐
🙁 ☹️ 😣

Food Intake:

TIME	FOOD	TRIGGERS/REACTION

Medications/Supplements

NAME	DOSAGE	TIME	SIDE EFFECTS/ COMMENTS

Notes:

Date:_____   Start:_____

Weather:_____   Water Intake: ⊔⊔⊔⊔⊔ ⊔⊔⊔⊔⊔
_____

Temperature:_____   Level of Pain
_____
No Pain   0 1 2 3 4 5 6 7 8 9 10   Severe Pain

Where does it hurt?	None—Mild—Moderate—Severe			
Back	☐	☐	☐	☐
Head	☐	☐	☐	☐
Neck	☐	☐	☐	☐
Shoulder	☐	☐	☐	☐
Elbow	☐	☐	☐	☐
Buttock	☐	☐	☐	☐
Knee	☐	☐	☐	☐
Hip	☐	☐	☐	☐
	☐	☐	☐	☐
	☐	☐	☐	☐

Interference of Pain on Sleep
_____

None   0 1 2 3 4 5 6 7 8 9 10   Significant

Fatigue
_____

None   0 1 2 3 4 5 6 7 8 9 10   Significant

Exercise
_____

Daily   0 1 2 3 4 5 6 7 8 9 10   No Exercise

Mood:

😊 🙂 😐
😟 ☹️ 😣

Food Intake:

TIME	FOOD	TRIGGERS/REACTION

Medications/Supplements

NAME	DOSAGE	TIME	SIDE EFFECTS/ COMMENTS

Notes:

Date:_____   Start:_____

Weather:_____   Water Intake: ⊽⊽⊽⊽⊽
_____   ⊽⊽⊽⊽⊽

Temperature:_____   Level of Pain
                      _____
                      No Pain   0 1 2 3 4 5 6 7 8 9 10   Severe Pain

Where does it hurt?	None—Mild—Moderate—Severe			
Back	☐	☐	☐	☐
Head	☐	☐	☐	☐
Neck	☐	☐	☐	☐
Shoulder	☐	☐	☐	☐
Elbow	☐	☐	☐	☐
Buttock	☐	☐	☐	☐
Knee	☐	☐	☐	☐
Hip	☐	☐	☐	☐
	☐	☐	☐	☐
	☐	☐	☐	☐

Interference of Pain on Sleep
_____
None   0 1 2 3 4 5 6 7 8 9 10   Significant

Fatigue
_____
None   0 1 2 3 4 5 6 7 8 9 10   Significant

Exercise
_____
Daily   0 1 2 3 4 5 6 7 8 9 10   No Exercise

Mood:
😊 🙂 😐
🙁 ☹️ 😣

Food Intake:

TIME	FOOD	TRIGGERS/REACTION

Medications/Supplements

NAME	DOSAGE	TIME	SIDE EFFECTS/ COMMENTS

Notes:

Date:_____   Start:_____

Weather:_____   Water Intake: ⊔⊔⊔⊔⊔
_____   ⊔⊔⊔⊔⊔

Temperature:_____   Level of Pain
                        No Pain   0 1 2 3 4 5 6 7 8 9 10   Severe Pain

Where does it hurt?	None—Mild—Moderate—Severe			
Back	☐	☐	☐	☐
Head	☐	☐	☐	☐
Neck	☐	☐	☐	☐
Shoulder	☐	☐	☐	☐
Elbow	☐	☐	☐	☐
Buttock	☐	☐	☐	☐
Knee	☐	☐	☐	☐
Hip	☐	☐	☐	☐
	☐	☐	☐	☐
	☐	☐	☐	☐

Interference of Pain on Sleep

None   0 1 2 3 4 5 6 7 8 9 10   Significant

Mood:

Fatigue

None   0 1 2 3 4 5 6 7 8 9 10   Significant

Exercise

Daily   0 1 2 3 4 5 6 7 8 9 10   No Exercise

Food Intake:

TIME	FOOD	TRIGGERS/REACTION

Medications/Supplements

NAME	DOSAGE	TIME	SIDE EFFECTS/ COMMENTS

Notes:

Date:_____   Start:_____

Weather:_____   Water Intake: ⊔⊔⊔⊔⊔
_____   ⊔⊔⊔⊔⊔

Temperature:_____   Level of Pain
_____
No Pain   0 1 2 3 4 5 6 7 8 9 10   Severe Pain

Where does it hurt?	None—Mild—Moderate—Severe
Back	☐ ☐ ☐ ☐
Head	☐ ☐ ☐ ☐
Neck	☐ ☐ ☐ ☐
Shoulder	☐ ☐ ☐ ☐
Elbow	☐ ☐ ☐ ☐
Buttock	☐ ☐ ☐ ☐
Knee	☐ ☐ ☐ ☐
Hip	☐ ☐ ☐ ☐
	☐ ☐ ☐ ☐
	☐ ☐ ☐ ☐

Interference of Pain on Sleep
_____
None   0 1 2 3 4 5 6 7 8 9 10   Significant

Fatigue
_____
None   0 1 2 3 4 5 6 7 8 9 10   Significant

Exercise
_____
Daily   0 1 2 3 4 5 6 7 8 9 10   No Exercise

Mood:
😊 🙂 😐
🙁 ☹️ 😣

Food Intake:

TIME	FOOD	TRIGGERS/REACTION

Medications/Supplements

NAME	DOSAGE	TIME	SIDE EFFECTS/ COMMENTS

Notes:

Date:_____   Start:_____

Weather:_____   Water Intake: ⊽⊽⊽⊽⊽
_____   ⊽⊽⊽⊽⊽

Temperature:_____   Level of Pain
_____
                        No Pain   0 1 2 3 4 5 6 7 8 9 10   Severe Pain

Where does it hurt?	None—Mild—Moderate—Severe			
Back	☐	☐	☐	☐
Head	☐	☐	☐	☐
Neck	☐	☐	☐	☐
Shoulder	☐	☐	☐	☐
Elbow	☐	☐	☐	☐
Buttock	☐	☐	☐	☐
Knee	☐	☐	☐	☐
Hip	☐	☐	☐	☐
	☐	☐	☐	☐
	☐	☐	☐	☐

Interference of Pain on Sleep
_____
None   0 1 2 3 4 5 6 7 8 9 10   Significant

Fatigue
_____
None   0 1 2 3 4 5 6 7 8 9 10   Significant

Exercise
_____
Daily   0 1 2 3 4 5 6 7 8 9 10   No Exercise

Mood:
☺ ☺ 😐
☹ ☹ 😣

Food Intake:

TIME	FOOD	TRIGGERS/REACTION

Medications/Supplements

NAME	DOSAGE	TIME	SIDE EFFECTS/ COMMENTS

Notes:

Date:_____ Start:_____

Weather:_____

_____ Water Intake:

Temperature:_____ Level of Pain

No Pain 0 1 2 3 4 5 6 7 8 9 10 Severe Pain

Where does it hurt?	None—Mild—Moderate—Severe			
Back	☐	☐	☐	☐
Head	☐	☐	☐	☐
Neck	☐	☐	☐	☐
Shoulder	☐	☐	☐	☐
Elbow	☐	☐	☐	☐
Buttock	☐	☐	☐	☐
Knee	☐	☐	☐	☐
Hip	☐	☐	☐	☐
	☐	☐	☐	☐
	☐	☐	☐	☐

Interference of Pain on Sleep

None   0 1 2 3 4 5 6 7 8 9 10   Significant

Mood:

Fatigue

None   0 1 2 3 4 5 6 7 8 9 10   Significant

Exercise

Daily   0 1 2 3 4 5 6 7 8 9 10   No Exercise

Food Intake:

TIME	FOOD	TRIGGERS/REACTION

Medications/Supplements

NAME	DOSAGE	TIME	SIDE EFFECTS/ COMMENTS

Notes:

Date:_____   Start:_____

Weather:_____   Water Intake: □□□□□ □□□□□
_____

Temperature:_____   Level of Pain
_____
No Pain   0 1 2 3 4 5 6 7 8 9 10   Severe Pain

Where does it hurt?	None—Mild—Moderate—Severe			
Back	□	□	□	□
Head	□	□	□	□
Neck	□	□	□	□
Shoulder	□	□	□	□
Elbow	□	□	□	□
Buttock	□	□	□	□
Knee	□	□	□	□
Hip	□	□	□	□
	□	□	□	□
	□	□	□	□

Interference of Pain on Sleep
_____
None   0 1 2 3 4 5 6 7 8 9 10   Significant

Mood:

Fatigue
_____
None   0 1 2 3 4 5 6 7 8 9 10   Significant

Exercise
_____
Daily   0 1 2 3 4 5 6 7 8 9 10   No Exercise

Food Intake:

TIME	FOOD	TRIGGERS/REACTION

Medications/Supplements

NAME	DOSAGE	TIME	SIDE EFFECTS/ COMMENTS

Notes:

Date:_____   Start:_____

Weather:_____   Water Intake: ▽▽▽▽▽
_____   ▽▽▽▽▽

Temperature:_____   Level of Pain
                          No Pain   0 1 2 3 4 5 6 7 8 9 10   Severe Pain

Where does it hurt?	None—Mild—Moderate—Severe			
Back	☐	☐	☐	☐
Head	☐	☐	☐	☐
Neck	☐	☐	☐	☐
Shoulder	☐	☐	☐	☐
Elbow	☐	☐	☐	☐
Buttock	☐	☐	☐	☐
Knee	☐	☐	☐	☐
Hip	☐	☐	☐	☐
	☐	☐	☐	☐
	☐	☐	☐	☐

Interference of Pain on Sleep
_____
None   0 1 2 3 4 5 6 7 8 9 10   Significant

Mood:

Fatigue
_____
None   0 1 2 3 4 5 6 7 8 9 10   Significant

Exercise
_____
Daily   0 1 2 3 4 5 6 7 8 9 10   No Exercise

Food Intake:

TIME	FOOD	TRIGGERS/REACTION

Medications/Supplements

NAME	DOSAGE	TIME	SIDE EFFECTS/ COMMENTS

Notes:

Date:_____   Start:_____

Weather:_____   Water Intake: ▽▽▽▽▽
_____   ▽▽▽▽▽

Temperature:_____   Level of Pain
                        _____
                        No Pain   0 1 2 3 4 5 6 7 8 9 10   Severe Pain

Where does it hurt?	None—Mild—Moderate—Severe			
Back	☐	☐	☐	☐
Head	☐	☐	☐	☐
Neck	☐	☐	☐	☐
Shoulder	☐	☐	☐	☐
Elbow	☐	☐	☐	☐
Buttock	☐	☐	☐	☐
Knee	☐	☐	☐	☐
Hip	☐	☐	☐	☐
	☐	☐	☐	☐
	☐	☐	☐	☐

Interference of Pain on Sleep
_____
None   0 1 2 3 4 5 6 7 8 9 10   Significant   Mood:

Fatigue
_____
None   0 1 2 3 4 5 6 7 8 9 10   Significant

Exercise
_____
Daily   0 1 2 3 4 5 6 7 8 9 10   No Exercise

Food Intake:

TIME	FOOD	TRIGGERS/REACTION

Medications/Supplements

NAME	DOSAGE	TIME	SIDE EFFECTS/ COMMENTS

Notes:

Date:_____   Start:_____

Weather:_____   Water Intake: ⊔⊔⊔⊔⊔
_____   ⊔⊔⊔⊔⊔

Temperature:_____   Level of Pain
_____
                             No Pain   0 1 2 3 4 5 6 7 8 9 10   Severe Pain

Where does it hurt?	None—Mild—Moderate—Severe			
Back	☐	☐	☐	☐
Head	☐	☐	☐	☐
Neck	☐	☐	☐	☐
Shoulder	☐	☐	☐	☐
Elbow	☐	☐	☐	☐
Buttock	☐	☐	☐	☐
Knee	☐	☐	☐	☐
Hip	☐	☐	☐	☐
	☐	☐	☐	☐
	☐	☐	☐	☐

Interference of Pain on Sleep
_____
None   0 1 2 3 4 5 6 7 8 9 10   Significant

Fatigue
_____
None   0 1 2 3 4 5 6 7 8 9 10   Significant

Exercise
_____
Daily   0 1 2 3 4 5 6 7 8 9 10   No Exercise

Mood:

Food Intake:

TIME	FOOD	TRIGGERS/REACTION

Medications/Supplements

NAME	DOSAGE	TIME	SIDE EFFECTS/ COMMENTS

Notes:

Date:_____   Start:_____

Weather:_____   Water Intake: ⬡⬡⬡⬡⬡
_____   ⬡⬡⬡⬡⬡

Temperature:_____   Level of Pain
_____
                        No Pain   0 1 2 3 4 5 6 7 8 9 10   Severe Pain

Where does it hurt?	None—Mild—Moderate—Severe			
Back	☐	☐	☐	☐
Head	☐	☐	☐	☐
Neck	☐	☐	☐	☐
Shoulder	☐	☐	☐	☐
Elbow	☐	☐	☐	☐
Buttock	☐	☐	☐	☐
Knee	☐	☐	☐	☐
Hip	☐	☐	☐	☐
	☐	☐	☐	☐
	☐	☐	☐	☐

Interference of Pain on Sleep
_____
None   0 1 2 3 4 5 6 7 8 9 10   Significant

Mood:

Fatigue
_____
None   0 1 2 3 4 5 6 7 8 9 10   Significant

Exercise
_____
Daily   0 1 2 3 4 5 6 7 8 9 10   No Exercise

Food Intake:

TIME	FOOD	TRIGGERS/REACTION

Medications/Supplements

NAME	DOSAGE	TIME	SIDE EFFECTS/ COMMENTS

Notes:

Date:_____   Start:_____

Weather:_____   Water Intake: ⛾⛾⛾⛾⛾
_____   ⛾⛾⛾⛾⛾

Temperature:_____   Level of Pain
_____
                        No Pain   0 1 2 3 4 5 6 7 8 9 10   Severe Pain

Where does it hurt?	None—Mild—Moderate—Severe
Back	☐ ☐ ☐ ☐
Head	☐ ☐ ☐ ☐
Neck	☐ ☐ ☐ ☐
Shoulder	☐ ☐ ☐ ☐
Elbow	☐ ☐ ☐ ☐
Buttock	☐ ☐ ☐ ☐
Knee	☐ ☐ ☐ ☐
Hip	☐ ☐ ☐ ☐
	☐ ☐ ☐ ☐
	☐ ☐ ☐ ☐

Interference of Pain on Sleep
_____
None   0 1 2 3 4 5 6 7 8 9 10   Significant

Mood:

Fatigue
_____
None   0 1 2 3 4 5 6 7 8 9 10   Significant

Exercise
_____
Daily   0 1 2 3 4 5 6 7 8 9 10   No Exercise

Food Intake:

TIME	FOOD	TRIGGERS/REACTION

Medications/Supplements

NAME	DOSAGE	TIME	SIDE EFFECTS/ COMMENTS

Notes:

Date:_____   Start:_____

Weather:_____   Water Intake: ⊽⊽⊽⊽⊽
_____   ⊽⊽⊽⊽⊽

Temperature:_____   Level of Pain
_____
                        No Pain   0 1 2 3 4 5 6 7 8 9 10   Severe Pain

Where does it hurt?	None—Mild—Moderate—Severe			
Back	☐	☐	☐	☐
Head	☐	☐	☐	☐
Neck	☐	☐	☐	☐
Shoulder	☐	☐	☐	☐
Elbow	☐	☐	☐	☐
Buttock	☐	☐	☐	☐
Knee	☐	☐	☐	☐
Hip	☐	☐	☐	☐
	☐	☐	☐	☐
	☐	☐	☐	☐

Interference of Pain on Sleep
_____
None   0 1 2 3 4 5 6 7 8 9 10   Significant

Fatigue
_____
None   0 1 2 3 4 5 6 7 8 9 10   Significant

Exercise
_____
Daily   0 1 2 3 4 5 6 7 8 9 10   No Exercise

Mood:

😊 🙂 😐

☹ ☹ 😣

Food Intake:

TIME	FOOD	TRIGGERS/REACTION

Medications/Supplements

NAME	DOSAGE	TIME	SIDE EFFECTS/ COMMENTS

Notes:

Date:_____ Start:_____

Weather:_____ Water Intake: ▽▽▽▽▽ ▽▽▽▽▽
_____

Temperature:_____ Level of Pain
_____
No Pain   0 1 2 3 4 5 6 7 8 9 10   Severe Pain

Where does it hurt?	None—Mild—Moderate—Severe			
Back	☐	☐	☐	☐
Head	☐	☐	☐	☐
Neck	☐	☐	☐	☐
Shoulder	☐	☐	☐	☐
Elbow	☐	☐	☐	☐
Buttock	☐	☐	☐	☐
Knee	☐	☐	☐	☐
Hip	☐	☐	☐	☐
	☐	☐	☐	☐
	☐	☐	☐	☐

Interference of Pain on Sleep
_____
None   0 1 2 3 4 5 6 7 8 9 10   Significant

Fatigue
_____
None   0 1 2 3 4 5 6 7 8 9 10   Significant

Exercise
_____
Daily   0 1 2 3 4 5 6 7 8 9 10   No Exercise

Mood:

☺ ☺ ☺
☹ ☹ ><

Food Intake:

TIME	FOOD	TRIGGERS/REACTION

Medications/Supplements

NAME	DOSAGE	TIME	SIDE EFFECTS/ COMMENTS

Notes:

Date:_____   Start:_____

Weather:_____   Water Intake: ⛶⛶⛶⛶⛶
_____   ⛶⛶⛶⛶⛶

Temperature:_____   Level of Pain
                        _____
                        No Pain   0 1 2 3 4 5 6 7 8 9 10   Severe Pain

Where does it hurt?	None—Mild—Moderate—Severe			
Back	☐	☐	☐	☐
Head	☐	☐	☐	☐
Neck	☐	☐	☐	☐
Shoulder	☐	☐	☐	☐
Elbow	☐	☐	☐	☐
Buttock	☐	☐	☐	☐
Knee	☐	☐	☐	☐
Hip	☐	☐	☐	☐
	☐	☐	☐	☐
	☐	☐	☐	☐

Interference of Pain on Sleep
_____
None   0 1 2 3 4 5 6 7 8 9 10   Significant

Fatigue
_____
None   0 1 2 3 4 5 6 7 8 9 10   Significant

Exercise
_____
Daily   0 1 2 3 4 5 6 7 8 9 10   No Exercise

Mood:

Food Intake:

TIME	FOOD	TRIGGERS/REACTION

Medications/Supplements

NAME	DOSAGE	TIME	SIDE EFFECTS/ COMMENTS

Notes:

Date:_____ Start:_____

Weather:_____
_____ Water Intake:

Temperature:_____ Level of Pain
_____
No Pain   0 1 2 3 4 5 6 7 8 9 10   Severe Pain

Where does it hurt?	None—Mild—Moderate—Severe			
Back	☐	☐	☐	☐
Head	☐	☐	☐	☐
Neck	☐	☐	☐	☐
Shoulder	☐	☐	☐	☐
Elbow	☐	☐	☐	☐
Buttock	☐	☐	☐	☐
Knee	☐	☐	☐	☐
Hip	☐	☐	☐	☐
	☐	☐	☐	☐
	☐	☐	☐	☐

Interference of Pain on Sleep
_____
None   0 1 2 3 4 5 6 7 8 9 10   Significant

Fatigue
_____
None   0 1 2 3 4 5 6 7 8 9 10   Significant

Exercise
_____
Daily   0 1 2 3 4 5 6 7 8 9 10   No Exercise

Mood:

Food Intake:

TIME	FOOD	TRIGGERS/REACTION

Medications/Supplements

NAME	DOSAGE	TIME	SIDE EFFECTS/ COMMENTS

Notes:

Date:_____   Start:_____

Weather:_____   Water Intake: ⊽⊽⊽⊽⊽
_____   ⊽⊽⊽⊽⊽

Temperature:_____   Level of Pain
_____
                       No Pain   0 1 2 3 4 5 6 7 8 9 10   Severe Pain

Where does it hurt?	None—Mild—Moderate—Severe			
Back	☐	☐	☐	☐
Head	☐	☐	☐	☐
Neck	☐	☐	☐	☐
Shoulder	☐	☐	☐	☐
Elbow	☐	☐	☐	☐
Buttock	☐	☐	☐	☐
Knee	☐	☐	☐	☐
Hip	☐	☐	☐	☐
	☐	☐	☐	☐
	☐	☐	☐	☐

Interference of Pain on Sleep
_____

None   0 1 2 3 4 5 6 7 8 9 10   Significant

Fatigue
_____

None   0 1 2 3 4 5 6 7 8 9 10   Significant

Exercise
_____

Daily   0 1 2 3 4 5 6 7 8 9 10   No Exercise

Mood:

☺ ☺ ☺
☹ ☹ ☹

Food Intake:

TIME	FOOD	TRIGGERS/REACTION

Medications/Supplements

NAME	DOSAGE	TIME	SIDE EFFECTS/ COMMENTS

Notes:

Date:_____   Start:_____

Weather:_____   Water Intake: ⊔⊔⊔⊔⊔
_____   ⊔⊔⊔⊔⊔

Temperature:_____   Level of Pain
_____
No Pain   0 1 2 3 4 5 6 7 8 9 10   Severe Pain

Where does it hurt?	None—Mild—Moderate—Severe
Back	☐ ☐ ☐ ☐
Head	☐ ☐ ☐ ☐
Neck	☐ ☐ ☐ ☐
Shoulder	☐ ☐ ☐ ☐
Elbow	☐ ☐ ☐ ☐
Buttock	☐ ☐ ☐ ☐
Knee	☐ ☐ ☐ ☐
Hip	☐ ☐ ☐ ☐
	☐ ☐ ☐ ☐
	☐ ☐ ☐ ☐

Interference of Pain on Sleep
_____
None   0 1 2 3 4 5 6 7 8 9 10   Significant

Fatigue
_____
None   0 1 2 3 4 5 6 7 8 9 10   Significant

Exercise
_____
Daily   0 1 2 3 4 5 6 7 8 9 10   No Exercise

Mood:
😊 🙂 😐
🙁 ☹️ 😣

Food Intake:

TIME	FOOD	TRIGGERS/REACTION

Medications/Supplements

NAME	DOSAGE	TIME	SIDE EFFECTS/ COMMENTS

Notes:

Date:_____   Start:_____

Weather:_____   Water Intake: [cups illustration: 5 + 5 cups]
_____

Temperature:_____   Level of Pain
_____
No Pain   0 1 2 3 4 5 6 7 8 9 10   Severe Pain

Where does it hurt?	None—Mild—Moderate—Severe			
Back	☐	☐	☐	☐
Head	☐	☐	☐	☐
Neck	☐	☐	☐	☐
Shoulder	☐	☐	☐	☐
Elbow	☐	☐	☐	☐
Buttock	☐	☐	☐	☐
Knee	☐	☐	☐	☐
Hip	☐	☐	☐	☐
	☐	☐	☐	☐
	☐	☐	☐	☐

Interference of Pain on Sleep
_____
None   0 1 2 3 4 5 6 7 8 9 10   Significant

Mood:

Fatigue
_____
None   0 1 2 3 4 5 6 7 8 9 10   Significant

Exercise
_____
Daily   0 1 2 3 4 5 6 7 8 9 10   No Exercise

Food Intake:

TIME	FOOD	TRIGGERS/REACTION

Medications/Supplements

NAME	DOSAGE	TIME	SIDE EFFECTS/ COMMENTS

Notes:

Date:_____   Start:_____

Weather:_____   Water Intake: ⊽⊽⊽⊽⊽
_____   ⊽⊽⊽⊽⊽

Temperature:_____   Level of Pain
_____
                        No Pain 0 1 2 3 4 5 6 7 8 9 10 Severe Pain

Where does it hurt?	None—Mild—Moderate—Severe			
Back	☐	☐	☐	☐
Head	☐	☐	☐	☐
Neck	☐	☐	☐	☐
Shoulder	☐	☐	☐	☐
Elbow	☐	☐	☐	☐
Buttock	☐	☐	☐	☐
Knee	☐	☐	☐	☐
Hip	☐	☐	☐	☐
	☐	☐	☐	☐
	☐	☐	☐	☐

Interference of Pain on Sleep
_____
None   0 1 2 3 4 5 6 7 8 9 10   Significant

Fatigue
_____
None   0 1 2 3 4 5 6 7 8 9 10   Significant

Exercise
_____
Daily   0 1 2 3 4 5 6 7 8 9 10   No Exercise

Mood:

☺ ☺ 😐
☹ ☹ ><

Food Intake:

TIME	FOOD	TRIGGERS/REACTION

Medications/Supplements

NAME	DOSAGE	TIME	SIDE EFFECTS/ COMMENTS

Notes:

Date:_____   Start:_____

Weather:_____   Water Intake: ⊔⊔⊔⊔⊔
_____   ⊔⊔⊔⊔⊔

Temperature:_____   Level of Pain
_____
No Pain   0 1 2 3 4 5 6 7 8 9 10   Severe Pain

Where does it hurt?	None—Mild—Moderate—Severe			
Back	☐	☐	☐	☐
Head	☐	☐	☐	☐
Neck	☐	☐	☐	☐
Shoulder	☐	☐	☐	☐
Elbow	☐	☐	☐	☐
Buttock	☐	☐	☐	☐
Knee	☐	☐	☐	☐
Hip	☐	☐	☐	☐
	☐	☐	☐	☐
	☐	☐	☐	☐

Interference of Pain on Sleep
_____
None   0 1 2 3 4 5 6 7 8 9 10   Significant

Fatigue
_____
None   0 1 2 3 4 5 6 7 8 9 10   Significant

Exercise
_____
Daily   0 1 2 3 4 5 6 7 8 9 10   No Exercise

Mood:
😊 🙂 😐
🙁 ☹️ 😣

Food Intake:

TIME	FOOD	TRIGGERS/REACTION

Medications/Supplements

NAME	DOSAGE	TIME	SIDE EFFECTS/ COMMENTS

Notes:

Date:_____   Start:_____

Weather:_____   Water Intake: ⊔⊔⊔⊔⊔
_____   ⊔⊔⊔⊔⊔

Temperature:_____   Level of Pain
                         _____
                         No Pain   0 1 2 3 4 5 6 7 8 9 10   Severe Pain

Where does it hurt?	None—Mild—Moderate—Severe
Back	☐ ☐ ☐ ☐
Head	☐ ☐ ☐ ☐
Neck	☐ ☐ ☐ ☐
Shoulder	☐ ☐ ☐ ☐
Elbow	☐ ☐ ☐ ☐
Buttock	☐ ☐ ☐ ☐
Knee	☐ ☐ ☐ ☐
Hip	☐ ☐ ☐ ☐
	☐ ☐ ☐ ☐
	☐ ☐ ☐ ☐

Interference of Pain on Sleep
_____
None   0 1 2 3 4 5 6 7 8 9 10   Significant

Fatigue
_____
None   0 1 2 3 4 5 6 7 8 9 10   Significant

Exercise
_____
Daily   0 1 2 3 4 5 6 7 8 9 10   No Exercise

Mood:

😊 🙂 😐

🙁 ☹ 😣

Food Intake:

TIME	FOOD	TRIGGERS/REACTION

Medications/Supplements

NAME	DOSAGE	TIME	SIDE EFFECTS/ COMMENTS

Notes:

Date:_____ Start:_____

Weather:_____

_____

Temperature:_____

Water Intake: ⊔⊔⊔⊔⊔
⊔⊔⊔⊔⊔

Level of Pain
_____

No Pain   0 1 2 3 4 5 6 7 8 9 10   Severe Pain

Where does it hurt?	None—Mild—Moderate—Severe			
Back	☐	☐	☐	☐
Head	☐	☐	☐	☐
Neck	☐	☐	☐	☐
Shoulder	☐	☐	☐	☐
Elbow	☐	☐	☐	☐
Buttock	☐	☐	☐	☐
Knee	☐	☐	☐	☐
Hip	☐	☐	☐	☐
	☐	☐	☐	☐
	☐	☐	☐	☐

Interference of Pain on Sleep
_____

None   0 1 2 3 4 5 6 7 8 9 10   Significant

Fatigue
_____

None   0 1 2 3 4 5 6 7 8 9 10   Significant

Exercise
_____

Daily   0 1 2 3 4 5 6 7 8 9 10   No Exercise

Mood:

Food Intake:

TIME	FOOD	TRIGGERS/REACTION

Medications/Supplements

NAME	DOSAGE	TIME	SIDE EFFECTS/ COMMENTS

Notes:

Date:_____   Start:_____

Weather:_____   Water Intake: ⊔⊔⊔⊔⊔
_____   ⊔⊔⊔⊔⊔

Temperature:_____   Level of Pain
                        _____
                        No Pain 0 1 2 3 4 5 6 7 8 9 10 Severe Pain

Where does it hurt?	None—Mild—Moderate—Severe			
Back	☐	☐	☐	☐
Head	☐	☐	☐	☐
Neck	☐	☐	☐	☐
Shoulder	☐	☐	☐	☐
Elbow	☐	☐	☐	☐
Buttock	☐	☐	☐	☐
Knee	☐	☐	☐	☐
Hip	☐	☐	☐	☐
	☐	☐	☐	☐
	☐	☐	☐	☐

Interference of Pain on Sleep
_____
None   0 1 2 3 4 5 6 7 8 9 10   Significant

Fatigue   Mood:
_____
None   0 1 2 3 4 5 6 7 8 9 10   Significant

Exercise
_____
Daily   0 1 2 3 4 5 6 7 8 9 10   No Exercise

Food Intake:

TIME	FOOD	TRIGGERS/REACTION

Medications/Supplements

NAME	DOSAGE	TIME	SIDE EFFECTS/ COMMENTS

Notes:

Date:_____ Start:_____

Weather:_____ Water Intake:
_____

Temperature:_____ Level of Pain
                       No Pain 0 1 2 3 4 5 6 7 8 9 10 Severe Pain

Where does it hurt?	None—Mild—Moderate—Severe
Back	☐ ☐ ☐ ☐
Head	☐ ☐ ☐ ☐
Neck	☐ ☐ ☐ ☐
Shoulder	☐ ☐ ☐ ☐
Elbow	☐ ☐ ☐ ☐
Buttock	☐ ☐ ☐ ☐
Knee	☐ ☐ ☐ ☐
Hip	☐ ☐ ☐ ☐
	☐ ☐ ☐ ☐
	☐ ☐ ☐ ☐

Interference of Pain on Sleep

None   0 1 2 3 4 5 6 7 8 9 10   Significant

Fatigue

None   0 1 2 3 4 5 6 7 8 9 10   Significant

Exercise

Daily   0 1 2 3 4 5 6 7 8 9 10   No Exercise

Mood:

Food Intake:

TIME	FOOD	TRIGGERS/REACTION

Medications/Supplements

NAME	DOSAGE	TIME	SIDE EFFECTS/ COMMENTS

Notes:

Date:_____ Start:_____

Weather:_____ Water Intake: ▽▽▽▽▽ ▽▽▽▽▽

_____

Temperature:_____ Level of Pain

No Pain 0 1 2 3 4 5 6 7 8 9 10 Severe Pain

Where does it hurt?	None—Mild—Moderate—Severe			
Back	☐	☐	☐	☐
Head	☐	☐	☐	☐
Neck	☐	☐	☐	☐
Shoulder	☐	☐	☐	☐
Elbow	☐	☐	☐	☐
Buttock	☐	☐	☐	☐
Knee	☐	☐	☐	☐
Hip	☐	☐	☐	☐
	☐	☐	☐	☐
	☐	☐	☐	☐

Interference of Pain on Sleep

Mood:

None   0 1 2 3 4 5 6 7 8 9 10   Significant

Fatigue

None   0 1 2 3 4 5 6 7 8 9 10   Significant

Exercise

Daily   0 1 2 3 4 5 6 7 8 9 10   No Exercise

Food Intake:

TIME	FOOD	TRIGGERS/REACTION

Medications/Supplements

NAME	DOSAGE	TIME	SIDE EFFECTS/ COMMENTS

Notes:

Date:_____   Start:_____

Weather:_____   Water Intake: ⊽⊽⊽⊽⊽
_____   ⊽⊽⊽⊽⊽

Temperature:_____   Level of Pain
_____
No Pain   0 1 2 3 4 5 6 7 8 9 10   Severe Pain

Where does it hurt?	None—Mild—Moderate—Severe			
Back	☐	☐	☐	☐
Head	☐	☐	☐	☐
Neck	☐	☐	☐	☐
Shoulder	☐	☐	☐	☐
Elbow	☐	☐	☐	☐
Buttock	☐	☐	☐	☐
Knee	☐	☐	☐	☐
Hip	☐	☐	☐	☐
	☐	☐	☐	☐
	☐	☐	☐	☐

Interference of Pain on Sleep
_____   Mood:
None   0 1 2 3 4 5 6 7 8 9 10   Significant

Fatigue
_____
None   0 1 2 3 4 5 6 7 8 9 10   Significant

Exercise
_____
Daily   0 1 2 3 4 5 6 7 8 9 10   No Exercise

Food Intake:

TIME	FOOD	TRIGGERS/REACTION

Medications/Supplements

NAME	DOSAGE	TIME	SIDE EFFECTS/ COMMENTS

Notes:

Date:_____   Start:_____

Weather:_____   Water Intake: ▽▽▽▽▽
_____   ▽▽▽▽▽

Temperature:_____   Level of Pain
_____
                       No Pain   0 1 2 3 4 5 6 7 8 9 10   Severe Pain

Where does it hurt?	None—Mild—Moderate—Severe			
Back	☐	☐	☐	☐
Head	☐	☐	☐	☐
Neck	☐	☐	☐	☐
Shoulder	☐	☐	☐	☐
Elbow	☐	☐	☐	☐
Buttock	☐	☐	☐	☐
Knee	☐	☐	☐	☐
Hip	☐	☐	☐	☐
	☐	☐	☐	☐
	☐	☐	☐	☐

Interference of Pain on Sleep
_____

None   0 1 2 3 4 5 6 7 8 9 10   Significant

Fatigue
_____

None   0 1 2 3 4 5 6 7 8 9 10   Significant

Exercise
_____

Daily   0 1 2 3 4 5 6 7 8 9 10   No Exercise

Mood:

Food Intake:

TIME	FOOD	TRIGGERS/REACTION

Medications/Supplements

NAME	DOSAGE	TIME	SIDE EFFECTS/ COMMENTS

Notes:

Date:_____   Start:_____

Weather:_____   Water Intake: ▽▽▽▽▽
_____   ▽▽▽▽▽

Temperature:_____   Level of Pain
_____
                      No Pain   0 1 2 3 4 5 6 7 8 9 10   Severe Pain

Where does it hurt?	None—Mild—Moderate—Severe			
Back	☐	☐	☐	☐
Head	☐	☐	☐	☐
Neck	☐	☐	☐	☐
Shoulder	☐	☐	☐	☐
Elbow	☐	☐	☐	☐
Buttock	☐	☐	☐	☐
Knee	☐	☐	☐	☐
Hip	☐	☐	☐	☐
	☐	☐	☐	☐
	☐	☐	☐	☐

Interference of Pain on Sleep
_____
None   0 1 2 3 4 5 6 7 8 9 10   Significant

Fatigue
_____
None   0 1 2 3 4 5 6 7 8 9 10   Significant

Exercise
_____
Daily   0 1 2 3 4 5 6 7 8 9 10   No Exercise

Mood:
☺ ☺ ☺
☹ ☹ ☹

Food Intake:

TIME	FOOD	TRIGGERS/REACTION

Medications/Supplements

NAME	DOSAGE	TIME	SIDE EFFECTS/ COMMENTS

Notes:

Date:_____ Start:_____

Weather:_____

_____ Water Intake: ⛆⛆⛆⛆⛆ ⛆⛆⛆⛆⛆

Temperature:_____

Level of Pain

No Pain 0 1 2 3 4 5 6 7 8 9 10 Severe Pain

Where does it hurt?	None—Mild—Moderate—Severe			
Back	☐	☐	☐	☐
Head	☐	☐	☐	☐
Neck	☐	☐	☐	☐
Shoulder	☐	☐	☐	☐
Elbow	☐	☐	☐	☐
Buttock	☐	☐	☐	☐
Knee	☐	☐	☐	☐
Hip	☐	☐	☐	☐
	☐	☐	☐	☐
	☐	☐	☐	☐

Interference of Pain on Sleep

None 0 1 2 3 4 5 6 7 8 9 10 Significant

Mood:

Fatigue

None 0 1 2 3 4 5 6 7 8 9 10 Significant

Exercise

Daily 0 1 2 3 4 5 6 7 8 9 10 No Exercise

Food Intake:

TIME	FOOD	TRIGGERS/REACTION

Medications/Supplements

NAME	DOSAGE	TIME	SIDE EFFECTS/ COMMENTS

Notes:

Date:_____   Start:_____

Weather:_____   Water Intake:
_____

Temperature:_____   Level of Pain

No Pain   0 1 2 3 4 5 6 7 8 9 10   Severe Pain

Where does it hurt?	None—Mild—Moderate—Severe			
Back	☐	☐	☐	☐
Head	☐	☐	☐	☐
Neck	☐	☐	☐	☐
Shoulder	☐	☐	☐	☐
Elbow	☐	☐	☐	☐
Buttock	☐	☐	☐	☐
Knee	☐	☐	☐	☐
Hip	☐	☐	☐	☐
	☐	☐	☐	☐
	☐	☐	☐	☐

Interference of Pain on Sleep

None   0 1 2 3 4 5 6 7 8 9 10   Significant

Fatigue

None   0 1 2 3 4 5 6 7 8 9 10   Significant

Exercise

Daily   0 1 2 3 4 5 6 7 8 9 10   No Exercise

Mood:

Food Intake:

TIME	FOOD	TRIGGERS/REACTION

Medications/Supplements

NAME	DOSAGE	TIME	SIDE EFFECTS/ COMMENTS

Notes:

Date:_____   Start:_____

Weather:_____   Water Intake: ⊔⊔⊔⊔⊔ ⊔⊔⊔⊔⊔
_____

Temperature:_____   ## Level of Pain

No Pain   0 1 2 3 4 5 6 7 8 9 10   Severe Pain

Where does it hurt?	None—Mild—Moderate—Severe			
Back	☐	☐	☐	☐
Head	☐	☐	☐	☐
Neck	☐	☐	☐	☐
Shoulder	☐	☐	☐	☐
Elbow	☐	☐	☐	☐
Buttock	☐	☐	☐	☐
Knee	☐	☐	☐	☐
Hip	☐	☐	☐	☐
	☐	☐	☐	☐
	☐	☐	☐	☐

Interference of Pain on Sleep

None   0 1 2 3 4 5 6 7 8 9 10   Significant

Fatigue

None   0 1 2 3 4 5 6 7 8 9 10   Significant

Exercise

Daily   0 1 2 3 4 5 6 7 8 9 10   No Exercise

Mood:

Food Intake:

TIME	FOOD	TRIGGERS/REACTION

Medications/Supplements

NAME	DOSAGE	TIME	SIDE EFFECTS/ COMMENTS

Notes:

Date:_____ Start:_____

Weather:_____ Water Intake: ⊽⊽⊽⊽⊽
_____ ⊽⊽⊽⊽⊽

Temperature:_____ Level of Pain
_____

No Pain 0 1 2 3 4 5 6 7 8 9 10 Severe Pain

Where does it hurt?	None—Mild—Moderate—Severe			
Back	☐	☐	☐	☐
Head	☐	☐	☐	☐
Neck	☐	☐	☐	☐
Shoulder	☐	☐	☐	☐
Elbow	☐	☐	☐	☐
Buttock	☐	☐	☐	☐
Knee	☐	☐	☐	☐
Hip	☐	☐	☐	☐
	☐	☐	☐	☐
	☐	☐	☐	☐

Interference of Pain on Sleep
_____

None   0 1 2 3 4 5 6 7 8 9 10   Significant

Fatigue
_____

None   0 1 2 3 4 5 6 7 8 9 10   Significant

Exercise
_____

Daily   0 1 2 3 4 5 6 7 8 9 10   No Exercise

Mood:

Food Intake:

TIME	FOOD	TRIGGERS/REACTION

Medications/Supplements

NAME	DOSAGE	TIME	SIDE EFFECTS/ COMMENTS

Notes:

Date:_____   Start:_____

Weather:_____   Water Intake: ⊔⊔⊔⊔⊔
_____   ⊔⊔⊔⊔⊔

Temperature:_____   Level of Pain
_____
                        No Pain   0 1 2 3 4 5 6 7 8 9 10   Severe Pain

Where does it hurt?	None—Mild—Moderate—Severe			
Back	☐	☐	☐	☐
Head	☐	☐	☐	☐
Neck	☐	☐	☐	☐
Shoulder	☐	☐	☐	☐
Elbow	☐	☐	☐	☐
Buttock	☐	☐	☐	☐
Knee	☐	☐	☐	☐
Hip	☐	☐	☐	☐
	☐	☐	☐	☐
	☐	☐	☐	☐

Interference of Pain on Sleep
_____
None   0 1 2 3 4 5 6 7 8 9 10   Significant

Fatigue
_____
None   0 1 2 3 4 5 6 7 8 9 10   Significant

Exercise
_____
Daily   0 1 2 3 4 5 6 7 8 9 10   No Exercise

Mood:
😊 🙂 😐
☹️ ☹️ 😖

Food Intake:

TIME	FOOD	TRIGGERS/REACTION

Medications/Supplements

NAME	DOSAGE	TIME	SIDE EFFECTS/ COMMENTS

Notes:

Date:_____   Start:_____

Weather:_____   Water Intake: ⊔⊔⊔⊔⊔
_____   ⊔⊔⊔⊔⊔

Temperature:_____   Level of Pain
_____
                       No Pain   0 1 2 3 4 5 6 7 8 9 10   Severe Pain

Where does it hurt?	None—Mild—Moderate—Severe			
Back	☐	☐	☐	☐
Head	☐	☐	☐	☐
Neck	☐	☐	☐	☐
Shoulder	☐	☐	☐	☐
Elbow	☐	☐	☐	☐
Buttock	☐	☐	☐	☐
Knee	☐	☐	☐	☐
Hip	☐	☐	☐	☐
	☐	☐	☐	☐
	☐	☐	☐	☐

Interference of Pain on Sleep
_____

None   0 1 2 3 4 5 6 7 8 9 10   Significant

Mood:

Fatigue
_____

None   0 1 2 3 4 5 6 7 8 9 10   Significant

Exercise
_____

Daily   0 1 2 3 4 5 6 7 8 9 10   No Exercise

Food Intake:

TIME	FOOD	TRIGGERS/REACTION

Medications/Supplements

NAME	DOSAGE	TIME	SIDE EFFECTS/ COMMENTS

Notes:

Date:_____ Start:_____

Weather:_____ Water Intake: ⊽⊽⊽⊽⊽
_____ ⊽⊽⊽⊽⊽

Temperature:_____ Level of Pain
_____

No Pain 0 1 2 3 4 5 6 7 8 9 10 Severe Pain

Where does it hurt?	None—Mild—Moderate—Severe
Back	☐ ☐ ☐ ☐
Head	☐ ☐ ☐ ☐
Neck	☐ ☐ ☐ ☐
Shoulder	☐ ☐ ☐ ☐
Elbow	☐ ☐ ☐ ☐
Buttock	☐ ☐ ☐ ☐
Knee	☐ ☐ ☐ ☐
Hip	☐ ☐ ☐ ☐
	☐ ☐ ☐ ☐
	☐ ☐ ☐ ☐

Interference of Pain on Sleep
_____

None   0 1 2 3 4 5 6 7 8 9 10   Significant

Mood:

Fatigue
_____

None   0 1 2 3 4 5 6 7 8 9 10   Significant

Exercise
_____

Daily   0 1 2 3 4 5 6 7 8 9 10   No Exercise

Food Intake:

TIME	FOOD	TRIGGERS/REACTION

Medications/Supplements

NAME	DOSAGE	TIME	SIDE EFFECTS/ COMMENTS

Notes:

Date:_____   Start:_____

Weather:_____   Water Intake: ⊔⊔⊔⊔⊔
_____   ⊔⊔⊔⊔⊔

Temperature:_____   Level of Pain
                              No Pain   0 1 2 3 4 5 6 7 8 9 10   Severe Pain

Where does it hurt?	None—Mild—Moderate—Severe			
Back	☐	☐	☐	☐
Head	☐	☐	☐	☐
Neck	☐	☐	☐	☐
Shoulder	☐	☐	☐	☐
Elbow	☐	☐	☐	☐
Buttock	☐	☐	☐	☐
Knee	☐	☐	☐	☐
Hip	☐	☐	☐	☐
	☐	☐	☐	☐
	☐	☐	☐	☐

Interference of Pain on Sleep

None   0 1 2 3 4 5 6 7 8 9 10   Significant

Fatigue

None   0 1 2 3 4 5 6 7 8 9 10   Significant

Exercise

Daily   0 1 2 3 4 5 6 7 8 9 10   No Exercise

Mood:
😊 🙂 😐
🙁 ☹️ 😣

Food Intake:

TIME	FOOD	TRIGGERS/REACTION

Medications/Supplements

NAME	DOSAGE	TIME	SIDE EFFECTS/ COMMENTS

Notes:

Date:_____ Start:_____

Weather:_____ Water Intake: ▽▽▽▽▽ ▽▽▽▽▽
_____

Temperature:_____ Level of Pain
_____
No Pain   0 1 2 3 4 5 6 7 8 9 10   Severe Pain

Where does it hurt?	None—Mild—Moderate—Severe			
Back	☐	☐	☐	☐
Head	☐	☐	☐	☐
Neck	☐	☐	☐	☐
Shoulder	☐	☐	☐	☐
Elbow	☐	☐	☐	☐
Buttock	☐	☐	☐	☐
Knee	☐	☐	☐	☐
Hip	☐	☐	☐	☐
	☐	☐	☐	☐
	☐	☐	☐	☐

Interference of Pain on Sleep
_____
None   0 1 2 3 4 5 6 7 8 9 10   Significant

Mood:

Fatigue
_____
None   0 1 2 3 4 5 6 7 8 9 10   Significant

Exercise
_____
Daily   0 1 2 3 4 5 6 7 8 9 10   No Exercise

Food Intake:

TIME	FOOD	TRIGGERS/REACTION

Medications/Supplements

NAME	DOSAGE	TIME	SIDE EFFECTS/ COMMENTS

Notes:

Date:_____   Start:_____

Weather:_____   Water Intake: ⊽⊽⊽⊽⊽
_____   ⊽⊽⊽⊽⊽

Temperature:_____   Level of Pain
_____

No Pain   0 1 2 3 4 5 6 7 8 9 10   Severe Pain

Where does it hurt?	None—Mild—Moderate—Severe			
Back	☐	☐	☐	☐
Head	☐	☐	☐	☐
Neck	☐	☐	☐	☐
Shoulder	☐	☐	☐	☐
Elbow	☐	☐	☐	☐
Buttock	☐	☐	☐	☐
Knee	☐	☐	☐	☐
Hip	☐	☐	☐	☐
	☐	☐	☐	☐
	☐	☐	☐	☐

Interference of Pain on Sleep
_____

None   0 1 2 3 4 5 6 7 8 9 10   Significant

Mood:

Fatigue
_____

None   0 1 2 3 4 5 6 7 8 9 10   Significant

Exercise
_____

Daily   0 1 2 3 4 5 6 7 8 9 10   No Exercise

Food Intake:

TIME	FOOD	TRIGGERS/REACTION

Medications/Supplements

NAME	DOSAGE	TIME	SIDE EFFECTS/ COMMENTS

Notes:

Date:_____   Start:_____

Weather:_____   Water Intake: ⊔⊔⊔⊔⊔
_____   ⊔⊔⊔⊔⊔

Temperature:_____   Level of Pain
_____
                         No Pain   0 1 2 3 4 5 6 7 8 9 10   Severe Pain

Where does it hurt?	None—Mild—Moderate—Severe
Back	☐ ☐ ☐ ☐
Head	☐ ☐ ☐ ☐
Neck	☐ ☐ ☐ ☐
Shoulder	☐ ☐ ☐ ☐
Elbow	☐ ☐ ☐ ☐
Buttock	☐ ☐ ☐ ☐
Knee	☐ ☐ ☐ ☐
Hip	☐ ☐ ☐ ☐
	☐ ☐ ☐ ☐
	☐ ☐ ☐ ☐

Interference of Pain on Sleep
_____
None   0 1 2 3 4 5 6 7 8 9 10   Significant

Fatigue
_____
None   0 1 2 3 4 5 6 7 8 9 10   Significant

Exercise
_____
Daily   0 1 2 3 4 5 6 7 8 9 10   No Exercise

Mood:
☺ ☺ ☹
☹ ☹ ☹

Food Intake:

TIME	FOOD	TRIGGERS/REACTION

Medications/Supplements

NAME	DOSAGE	TIME	SIDE EFFECTS/ COMMENTS

Notes:

Date:_____   Start:_____

Weather:_____   Water Intake: ▽▽▽▽▽
_____   ▽▽▽▽▽

Temperature:_____   Level of Pain
_____
                              No Pain   0 1 2 3 4 5 6 7 8 9 10   Severe Pain

Where does it hurt?	None—Mild—Moderate—Severe			
Back	☐	☐	☐	☐
Head	☐	☐	☐	☐
Neck	☐	☐	☐	☐
Shoulder	☐	☐	☐	☐
Elbow	☐	☐	☐	☐
Buttock	☐	☐	☐	☐
Knee	☐	☐	☐	☐
Hip	☐	☐	☐	☐
	☐	☐	☐	☐
	☐	☐	☐	☐

Interference of Pain on Sleep
_____
None   0 1 2 3 4 5 6 7 8 9 10   Significant

Fatigue
_____
None   0 1 2 3 4 5 6 7 8 9 10   Significant

Exercise
_____
Daily   0 1 2 3 4 5 6 7 8 9 10   No Exercise

Mood:
😊 🙂 😐
🙁 ☹️ 😣

Food Intake:

TIME	FOOD	TRIGGERS/REACTION

Medications/Supplements

NAME	DOSAGE	TIME	SIDE EFFECTS/ COMMENTS

Notes:

Date:_____ Start:_____

Weather:_____ Water Intake: ⊽⊽⊽⊽⊽
_____ ⊽⊽⊽⊽⊽

Temperature:_____ Level of Pain
_____
No Pain 0 1 2 3 4 5 6 7 8 9 10 Severe Pain

Where does it hurt?	None—Mild—Moderate—Severe			
Back	☐	☐	☐	☐
Head	☐	☐	☐	☐
Neck	☐	☐	☐	☐
Shoulder	☐	☐	☐	☐
Elbow	☐	☐	☐	☐
Buttock	☐	☐	☐	☐
Knee	☐	☐	☐	☐
Hip	☐	☐	☐	☐
	☐	☐	☐	☐
	☐	☐	☐	☐

Interference of Pain on Sleep
_____
None   0 1 2 3 4 5 6 7 8 9 10   Significant

Fatigue
_____
None   0 1 2 3 4 5 6 7 8 9 10   Significant

Exercise
_____
Daily   0 1 2 3 4 5 6 7 8 9 10   No Exercise

Mood:

😊 🙂 😐
☹ 😞 😣

Food Intake:

TIME	FOOD	TRIGGERS/REACTION

Medications/Supplements

NAME	DOSAGE	TIME	SIDE EFFECTS/ COMMENTS

Notes:

Date:_____   Start:_____

Weather:_____   Water Intake: ⊽⊽⊽⊽⊽
_____   ⊽⊽⊽⊽⊽

Temperature:_____   Level of Pain
_____
                        No Pain 0 1 2 3 4 5 6 7 8 9 10 Severe Pain

Where does it hurt?	None—Mild—Moderate—Severe			
Back	☐	☐	☐	☐
Head	☐	☐	☐	☐
Neck	☐	☐	☐	☐
Shoulder	☐	☐	☐	☐
Elbow	☐	☐	☐	☐
Buttock	☐	☐	☐	☐
Knee	☐	☐	☐	☐
Hip	☐	☐	☐	☐
	☐	☐	☐	☐
	☐	☐	☐	☐

Interference of Pain on Sleep

None   0 1 2 3 4 5 6 7 8 9 10   Significant

Fatigue

None   0 1 2 3 4 5 6 7 8 9 10   Significant

Exercise

Daily   0 1 2 3 4 5 6 7 8 9 10   No Exercise

Mood:

Food Intake:

TIME	FOOD	TRIGGERS/REACTION

Medications/Supplements

NAME	DOSAGE	TIME	SIDE EFFECTS/ COMMENTS

Notes:

Date:_____   Start:_____

Weather:_____   Water Intake: ▽▽▽▽▽
_____   ▽▽▽▽▽

Temperature:_____   Level of Pain
_____   No Pain 0 1 2 3 4 5 6 7 8 9 10 Severe Pain

Where does it hurt?	None—Mild—Moderate—Severe			
Back	☐	☐	☐	☐
Head	☐	☐	☐	☐
Neck	☐	☐	☐	☐
Shoulder	☐	☐	☐	☐
Elbow	☐	☐	☐	☐
Buttock	☐	☐	☐	☐
Knee	☐	☐	☐	☐
Hip	☐	☐	☐	☐
	☐	☐	☐	☐
	☐	☐	☐	☐

Interference of Pain on Sleep

None   0 1 2 3 4 5 6 7 8 9 10   Significant

Mood:

Fatigue

None   0 1 2 3 4 5 6 7 8 9 10   Significant

Exercise

Daily   0 1 2 3 4 5 6 7 8 9 10   No Exercise

Food Intake:

TIME	FOOD	TRIGGERS/REACTION

Medications/Supplements

NAME	DOSAGE	TIME	SIDE EFFECTS/ COMMENTS

Notes:

Date:_____   Start:_____

Weather:_____   Water Intake: ▽▽▽▽▽
_____   ▽▽▽▽▽

Temperature:_____   Level of Pain
                        _____
                        No Pain   0 1 2 3 4 5 6 7 8 9 10   Severe Pain

Where does it hurt?	None—Mild—Moderate—Severe			
Back	☐	☐	☐	☐
Head	☐	☐	☐	☐
Neck	☐	☐	☐	☐
Shoulder	☐	☐	☐	☐
Elbow	☐	☐	☐	☐
Buttock	☐	☐	☐	☐
Knee	☐	☐	☐	☐
Hip	☐	☐	☐	☐
	☐	☐	☐	☐
	☐	☐	☐	☐

Interference of Pain on Sleep
_____
None   0 1 2 3 4 5 6 7 8 9 10   Significant

Mood:

Fatigue
_____
None   0 1 2 3 4 5 6 7 8 9 10   Significant

Exercise
_____
Daily   0 1 2 3 4 5 6 7 8 9 10   No Exercise

Food Intake:

TIME	FOOD	TRIGGERS/REACTION

Medications/Supplements

NAME	DOSAGE	TIME	SIDE EFFECTS/ COMMENTS

Notes:

Date:_____   Start:_____

Weather:_____   Water Intake: ☐☐☐☐☐
_____   ☐☐☐☐☐

Temperature:_____   Level of Pain
_____
No Pain   0 1 2 3 4 5 6 7 8 9 10   Severe Pain

Where does it hurt?	None—Mild—Moderate—Severe			
Back	☐	☐	☐	☐
Head	☐	☐	☐	☐
Neck	☐	☐	☐	☐
Shoulder	☐	☐	☐	☐
Elbow	☐	☐	☐	☐
Buttock	☐	☐	☐	☐
Knee	☐	☐	☐	☐
Hip	☐	☐	☐	☐
	☐	☐	☐	☐
	☐	☐	☐	☐

Interference of Pain on Sleep
_____

None   0 1 2 3 4 5 6 7 8 9 10   Significant

Mood:

Fatigue
_____

None   0 1 2 3 4 5 6 7 8 9 10   Significant

Exercise
_____

Daily   0 1 2 3 4 5 6 7 8 9 10   No Exercise

Food Intake:

TIME	FOOD	TRIGGERS/REACTION

Medications/Supplements

NAME	DOSAGE	TIME	SIDE EFFECTS/ COMMENTS

Notes:

Date:_____   Start:_____

Weather:_____   Water Intake: ⊽⊽⊽⊽⊽
_____   ⊽⊽⊽⊽⊽

Temperature:_____   Level of Pain
_____

No Pain   0 1 2 3 4 5 6 7 8 9 10   Severe Pain

Where does it hurt?	None—Mild—Moderate—Severe			
Back	☐	☐	☐	☐
Head	☐	☐	☐	☐
Neck	☐	☐	☐	☐
Shoulder	☐	☐	☐	☐
Elbow	☐	☐	☐	☐
Buttock	☐	☐	☐	☐
Knee	☐	☐	☐	☐
Hip	☐	☐	☐	☐
	☐	☐	☐	☐
	☐	☐	☐	☐

Interference of Pain on Sleep
_____

None   0 1 2 3 4 5 6 7 8 9 10   Significant

Mood:

Fatigue
_____

None   0 1 2 3 4 5 6 7 8 9 10   Significant

Exercise
_____

Daily   0 1 2 3 4 5 6 7 8 9 10   No Exercise

Food Intake:

TIME	FOOD	TRIGGERS/REACTION

Medications/Supplements

NAME	DOSAGE	TIME	SIDE EFFECTS/ COMMENTS

Notes:

Date:_____ Start:_____

Weather:_____ Water Intake: ⊽⊽⊽⊽⊽
_____ ⊽⊽⊽⊽⊽

Temperature:_____ Level of Pain
_____
No Pain 0 1 2 3 4 5 6 7 8 9 10 Severe Pain

Where does it hurt?	None—Mild—Moderate—Severe			
Back	☐	☐	☐	☐
Head	☐	☐	☐	☐
Neck	☐	☐	☐	☐
Shoulder	☐	☐	☐	☐
Elbow	☐	☐	☐	☐
Buttock	☐	☐	☐	☐
Knee	☐	☐	☐	☐
Hip	☐	☐	☐	☐
	☐	☐	☐	☐
	☐	☐	☐	☐

Interference of Pain on Sleep
_____
None 0 1 2 3 4 5 6 7 8 9 10 Significant

Fatigue
_____
None 0 1 2 3 4 5 6 7 8 9 10 Significant

Exercise
_____
Daily 0 1 2 3 4 5 6 7 8 9 10 No Exercise

Mood:

Food Intake:

TIME	FOOD	TRIGGERS/REACTION

Medications/Supplements

NAME	DOSAGE	TIME	SIDE EFFECTS/ COMMENTS

Notes:

Date:_____ Start:_____

Weather:_____ Water Intake: ⛾⛾⛾⛾⛾
_____ ⛾⛾⛾⛾⛾

Temperature:_____ Level of Pain
_____
No Pain   0 1 2 3 4 5 6 7 8 9 10   Severe Pain

Where does it hurt?	None—Mild—Moderate—Severe			
Back	☐	☐	☐	☐
Head	☐	☐	☐	☐
Neck	☐	☐	☐	☐
Shoulder	☐	☐	☐	☐
Elbow	☐	☐	☐	☐
Buttock	☐	☐	☐	☐
Knee	☐	☐	☐	☐
Hip	☐	☐	☐	☐
	☐	☐	☐	☐
	☐	☐	☐	☐

Interference of Pain on Sleep
_____
None   0 1 2 3 4 5 6 7 8 9 10   Significant

Fatigue
_____
None   0 1 2 3 4 5 6 7 8 9 10   Significant

Exercise
_____
Daily   0 1 2 3 4 5 6 7 8 9 10   No Exercise

Mood:

Food Intake:

TIME	FOOD	TRIGGERS/REACTION

Medications/Supplements

NAME	DOSAGE	TIME	SIDE EFFECTS/ COMMENTS

Notes:

Date:_____ Start:_____

Weather:_____ Water Intake:
_____

Temperature:_____ Level of Pain
_____
No Pain   0 1 2 3 4 5 6 7 8 9 10   Severe Pain

Where does it hurt?	None—Mild—Moderate—Severe			
Back	☐	☐	☐	☐
Head	☐	☐	☐	☐
Neck	☐	☐	☐	☐
Shoulder	☐	☐	☐	☐
Elbow	☐	☐	☐	☐
Buttock	☐	☐	☐	☐
Knee	☐	☐	☐	☐
Hip	☐	☐	☐	☐
	☐	☐	☐	☐
	☐	☐	☐	☐

Interference of Pain on Sleep
_____
None   0 1 2 3 4 5 6 7 8 9 10   Significant

Mood:

Fatigue
_____
None   0 1 2 3 4 5 6 7 8 9 10   Significant

Exercise
_____
Daily   0 1 2 3 4 5 6 7 8 9 10   No Exercise

Food Intake:

TIME	FOOD	TRIGGERS/REACTION

Medications/Supplements

NAME	DOSAGE	TIME	SIDE EFFECTS/ COMMENTS

Notes:

Made in the USA
Coppell, TX
17 March 2023

14388292R00069